EVERYTHING ABOUT POLYCYTHEMIA VERA

A Complete Guide For Patients, Caregivers, And Healthcare Professionals - Causes, Symptoms, Diagnosis, Treatment, Coping Strategies, And More

DR. CADE JOSUE

Table of Contents

DISCLAIMER

The information provided in this book is for general informational purposes only. It is not intended as medical advice, diagnosis, or treatment.

The content of this book should not be considered a substitute for professional medical advice. Readers should consult with a qualified healthcare provider for diagnosis and treatment of any medical conditions they have.

While every effort has been made to ensure the accuracy and completeness of the information presented, the author makes no representations or warranties of any kind, express or implied, about the completeness, accuracy, reliability, suitability, or availability with respect to the information, contained in this book.

The author disclaims any responsibility for any loss or damage resulting from reliance on the information provided in this book. References to individuals, products, websites, organizations, or other names are for informational purposes only and do not imply endorsement.

By reading this book, readers acknowledge that they are responsible for their own health decisions and should seek appropriate medical advice when necessary.

ABOUT THIS BOOK

"Everything About Polycythemia Vera" serves as an essential reference for patients, researchers, and healthcare professionals who are interested in gaining a thorough understanding of this uncommon yet consequential blood disorder. This book functions as an all-encompassing manual, addressing all aspects of Polycythemia Vera (PV), including its fundamental definition, advanced therapeutic approaches, and potential avenues for future research.

The introductory section offers a concise synopsis, establishing the foundation for a comprehensive investigation of PV. It provides an overview of the book's aims and prepares the reader for the abundance of information that will ensue.

The following chapters provide a comprehensive analysis of PV, commencing with an introductory section that clarifies its pathophysiology, epidemiology, and etiology. The discourse surrounding the causes and risk factors of the disease enhances comprehension by illuminating its multifactorial nature.

The symptoms and indications, which are frequently enigmatic in nature, are thoroughly clarified, which aids in the prompt identification and diagnosis. The sections about diagnostic modalities, such as bone marrow biopsy, blood tests, and imaging techniques, furnish medical professionals with the essential resources to conduct precise evaluations.

A thorough examination of treatment alternatives is conducted, including phlebotomy, pharmaceuticals, surgical procedures, and adjustments to one's lifestyle. Every approach is thoroughly analyzed, taking into account its effectiveness, recommended uses, and possible adverse reactions.

It is crucial to comprehend the intricacies linked to PV to implement efficient management strategies. This book explores the complexities associated with blood coagulation, propensity for hemorrhage, splenic enlargement, myelofibrosis, and the concerning progression to leukemia.

The segment about the management of PV emphasizes the criticality of proactive follow-up care, namely the role that supportive therapies and routine blood count monitoring play in maximizing patient outcomes.

The ability to forecast outcomes is critical for informing therapeutic choices and establishing practical anticipations. The sections about life expectancy, quality of life, and prognostic factors provide indispensable knowledge regarding the progression of the disease.

In addition, this book delves into current research initiatives and prospective trajectories, encompassing clinical trials and developments in therapeutic modalities. Healthcare providers can ensure patients receive the most advanced care possible by remaining updated on emerging therapies.

In conclusion, "Everything About Polycythemia Vera" is a seminal piece of literature in the field, providing an exhaustive compilation of vital information for patients and healthcare professionals. The resource's forward-looking perspective, evidence-based approach, and meticulous attention to detail render it an essential tool in the management of PV.

CHAPTER ONE

An Overview Of Polycythemia Vera

Polycythemia Vera (PV) is an uncommon chronic blood disorder distinguished by platelet, white blood, and red blood cell overproduction in the bone marrow (erythrocytosis). This condition is classified as a myeloproliferative neoplasm, which comprises a cluster of disorders characterized by an excessive proliferation of bone marrow cells that results in an elevation of blood cell counts.

A Synopsis Of Polycythemia Vera

PV is attributed to a genetic mutation that occurs specifically in the Janus kinase 2 (JAK2) gene of bone marrow progenitor cells. Due to the uncontrolled proliferation of blood cells caused by this mutation, platelets, white blood cells, and red blood cells are significantly increased in number. The heightened generation of these cells results in a viscous circulation, thereby augmenting the likelihood of blood clotting and additional complications.

PV is generally a disease with a gradual progression and extended periods of asymptomatic status. It can, however, result in severe complications including blood clotting, stroke, myocardial infarction, and leukemia if left untreated.

Contributing Factors And Risk Elements

Although the precise etiology of PV remains unknown, it is hypothesized that it arises from a complex interplay of genetic and environmental influences. The JAK2 mutation, which is present in approximately 95% of cases, is the most prevalent genetic abnormality linked to PV. This mutation induces the activation of signaling pathways that facilitate excessive blood cell production.

Although PV can manifest at any stage of life, elderly adults. are diagnosed with it more frequently, with a median age of diagnosis of approximately 60 years. Men also have a marginally higher incidence of PV than women.

The following are potential risk factors for PV:

1. A familial history of PV or other myeloproliferative disorders elevates the likelihood of an individual developing this particular condition.

2. Prolonged exposure to specific contaminants, including benzene, a chemical commonly encountered in industrial environments, has the potential to elevate the likelihood of developing PV.

3. PV is diagnosed with greater frequency in the elderly, specifically in those who have surpassed the age of 60.

4. Gender: The incidence of PV is marginally higher among men compared to women.

Signals And Symptoms

The symptoms of PV may be nonspecific and can vary considerably between patients, making diagnosis difficult. Common indications and symptoms of PV include the following:

1. Headaches may be a common occurrence for individuals with PV as a result of elevated blood viscosity.

2. Excessive blood cell production can result in both fatigue and frailty.

3. A decrease in blood supply to the brain may result in the sensation of vertigo or lightheadedness.

4. Pulmonary obstruction: Raised blood pressure can hinder the delivery of oxygen to various tissues, leading to the development of dyspnea.

5. Pruritus, or itching, is a symptom that certain individuals diagnosed with PV may encounter, especially following a heated bath or shower.

6. Erythromelalgia, characterized by a discoloration of the skin that is reddish or purplish in hue, may result from an increase in blood flow to small blood vessels. This condition is most prevalent in the hands and feet.

7. Splenomegaly, an enlargement of the spleen, may occur as a result of an overabundance of blood cells.

The Diagnosis

A combination of medical history, physical examination, and laboratory tests are utilized to diagnose PV. The diagnostic procedure typically encompasses the subsequent stages:

1. During the physical examination and medical history review, the healthcare provider will inquire about the patient's symptoms, medical history, and any blood disorders that may have run in the family. Symptoms such as reddish skin discoloration or an enlarged spleen may be detected during a physical examination.

2. Blood investigations are an essential component in the diagnosis of PV. An elevated count of red blood cells, white blood cells, and platelets is indicated by a complete blood count (CBC). Furthermore, distinctive alterations in the visual characteristics of blood cells might be detected via peripheral blood smear.

3. Testing for the JAK2 mutation can assist in confirming the diagnosis of PV, as this mutation is observed in the majority of cases. Blood is typically drawn for this purpose.

4. Bone marrow biopsy: A bone marrow biopsy may be performed in certain instances to investigate the cells of the bone marrow for PV-specific abnormalities. A catheter is inserted into the bone marrow to obtain a minute sample for subsequent analysis.

5. Depending on the specific circumstances, imaging studies (e.g., MRI, ultrasound) and other diagnostic procedures may be administered to evaluate for complications such as enlarged organs or blood blockages.

Treatment for PV, once diagnosed, seeks to manage symptoms and reduce the risk of complications. This may encompass pharmacological interventions aimed at decreasing the number of red blood cells, such as hydroxyurea or interferon-alpha, in addition to preventative measures against blood clotting, including phlebotomy or aspirin therapy. Continuous monitoring is critical for determining the course of a disease and modifying treatment accordingly.

CHAPTER TWO

Tests Of The Blood For Polycythemia Vera

The utilization of blood tests is critical in the diagnosis of PV. Essential testing consists of:

• Complete Blood Count (CBC): Determines the platelet, red blood, and white blood cell counts of the blood. Typically, the red blood cell concentration is increased in PV.

Erythropoietin (EPO) is a hormone that is secreted by the kidneys and is responsible for promoting the synthesis of red blood cells. EPO levels are diminished in PV because red blood cells are produced by the body in the absence of EPO signals.

• Peripheral Blood Smear: The size, shape, and quantity of blood cells are evaluated by examining a blood sample under a microscope. Red blood cells may appear aberrant or congested in PV.

Genetic tests can detect PV through mutations in the JAK2, CALR, or MPL genes, which are frequently linked to the condition. Molecular genetics can verify the existence of these mutations.

Anatomical Bone Marrow Biopsy

A bone marrow biopsy may be performed to assess the extent of bone marrow involvement and confirm a diagnosis of PV. As part of this procedure:

• Typically, a minute specimen of bone marrow is isolated, originating from the hip bone.

• The sample is examined under a microscope to determine the quantity and morphology of blood cells.

• A diagnosis of PV is supported by the presence of an increased number of red blood cells and alterations in other blood cell types.

Imaging Examinations

For the evaluation of PV complications such as blood blockages or enlarged organs, imaging techniques may be utilized. Frequent imaging modalities consist of:

To evaluate blood flow and identify blood obstructions in capillaries or arteries, ultrasound is utilized.

• Computed Tomography (CT) or Magnetic Resonance Imaging (MRI) Scan: These imaging modalities can detect enlarged organs, including the spleen or liver, that may manifest as a consequence of heightened blood cell generation in PV.

1. Echocardiogram: This diagnostic procedure evaluates cardiac functionality and identifies irregularities, including myocardium or indications of strain resulting from elevated blood viscosity.

Alternatives To Treatment

Phlebotomy Involves:

Blood removal, or phlebotomy, is the principal therapeutic approach for PV. The primary objective is to suppress the number of erythrocytes present in the circulation to avert potential complications linked to thrombosis. Ahead of phlebotomy:

• Typically, a specific volume of blood is extracted from the body via a vein located in the arm.

• To maintain a desired range of hematocrit (the proportion of red blood cells in the blood), routine phlebotomy sessions may be required. Pneubotomy is typically conducted periodically thereafter, until the hematocrit level returns to normal, to mitigate the risk of recurrence.

Pharmaceutical Agents:

Cytoreductive therapy involves the administration of pharmaceutical agents like hydroxyurea or interferon-alpha to inhibit the erythrocyte sedimentation rate (PV) in the bone marrow, especially when phlebotomy proves inadequate in controlling the condition. A low dose of aspirin might be advised to decrease the likelihood of developing blood clotting.

Symptom And Complication Management

• Hydration: Adequate hydration reduces the risk of blood clotting and helps maintain blood flow.

• Avoiding Alcohol and Smoking: Excessive alcohol and smoking can increase the risk of complications associated with PV.

Patients diagnosed with PV necessitate routine follow-up consultations and blood analyses to assess blood cell counts, organ functionality, treatment efficacy, and treatment alternatives.

In conclusion, a holistic approach is necessary for the diagnosis, treatment, and management of polycythemia vera. Phlebotomy, blood tests, bone marrow biopsies, imaging tests, management with medications, and lifestyle modifications are all integral elements in the prevention of complications and effective management of this condition. Improving outcomes and quality of life for individuals with PV requires timely detection and effective treatment.

Pharmaceutical Medications

• Phlebotomy: Therapeutic phlebotomy, which removes surplus blood from the body to decrease the concentration of red blood cells and the danger of coagulation, is the primary treatment for

PV. Regular occurrences of this procedure are observed until hematocrit levels reach a state of stability.

• Medications to inhibit blood cell production: Certain medications, including hydroxyurea, interferon-alpha, and ruxolitinib, may be prescribed to assist in the reduction of blood cell concentrations. These medications function by inhibiting the erythrocyte production in the bone marrow.

A low dose of aspirin may be suggested as a preventative measure against blood clotting through the inhibition of platelet aggregation. Nevertheless, extreme caution should be exercised when administering it, particularly in those who are susceptible to complications involving hemorrhage.

• Surgical intervention may be necessary in certain instances to manage complications or reduce the risk of thrombosis in patients with PV. Spenectomy, an example of such a procedure, entails the excision of the spleen. Patients diagnosed with PV who exhibit symptomatic splenomegaly (spleen enlargement) or who fail to respond satisfactorily to alternative therapeutic interventions may warrant a splenectomy.

• Thrombectomy, an alternative surgical procedure, entails the excision of blood clots from the afflicted blood vessels. In situations involving substantial blood flow impairment or severe thrombosis, this procedure may be executed.

CHAPTER THREE

Lifestyle Alterations

• Hydration: Individuals with PV must maintain adequate hydration to prevent the blood from becoming excessively viscous. Adequate hydration can aid in blood circulation maintenance and decrease the likelihood of thrombus formation.

• Tobacco cessation: Individuals with PV who smoke are at an increased risk of developing blood clotting and cardiovascular complications. Cessation of smoking is thus highly advised.

Participating in consistent physical activity can aid in the enhancement of circulation and the mitigation of blood clot formation. Before beginning any exercise regimen, individuals with PV should consult their healthcare provider to ensure that it is safe for them.

The Cause Of Complications

Thrombosis is a highly consequential complication of PV characterized by the development of blood clotting in vessels or arteries across the entirety of the organism. Critical conditions such as strokes, myocardial infarctions, and pulmonary embolisms may result from these blockages.

• Bleeding: While less prevalent compared to thrombotic events, individuals with PV are susceptible to developing complications related to bleeding, especially if they are regular phlebotomists or are prescribed anticoagulant medications. Bleeding can manifest either spontaneously or in response to an injury sustained during medical procedures.

• Myelofibrosis: PV may occasionally advance to myelofibrosis, an advanced form of bone marrow disorder distinguished by the fibrous deposition on top of healthy marrow. Anemia, fatigue, and an enlarged spleen may result from this.

Clots In Blood

Arterial thrombosis is a pathological condition characterized by the occlusion of blood flow to critical organs, including the brain (painful strokes), heart (atrial fibrillation), and extremities (peripheral artery disease), by clots that develop in the arteries. Irregular blood vessel thrombosis is a critical complication of PV that demands immediate medical intervention.

• Venous thrombosis: The formation of blood clots within the vessels can give rise to various complications, including pulmonary embolism (PE) and deep vein thrombosis (DVT). DVT is characterized by the formation of a clot in a deep vein, typically in the legs; PE is characterized by the travel of a clot to the lungs, where it can rupture and cause potentially fatal respiratory complications.

• Thrombotic microangiopathy: Feasibly uncommon, PV patients may manifest thrombotic microangiopathy, a pathological state distinguished by the development of minute blood clots within the capillaries. This can result in dysfunction and injury to organs, especially the kidneys and brain.

In essence, the control of polycythemia vera necessitates a comprehensive strategy that targets the reduction of red blood cell counts, the prevention of clotting-related complications, and the resolution of associated health issues.

To enhance prognoses or manage complications, this uncommon blood disorder is often treated with surgical interventions or lifestyle modifications. Medications and lifestyle modifications are common components of this treatment regimen.

Experiencing Bleeding Due To Polycythemia Vera

Bleeding is one of the complications that may arise as a result of PV. Although an overproduction of red blood cells is a defining feature of PV, these cells may not operate ordinarily. An elevated red blood cell count can cause an increase in blood viscosity, potentially resulting in compromised circulation and subsequent tissue injury and hemorrhaging. Furthermore, compromised platelet function, which is a prevalent characteristic of PV, may additionally exacerbate the propensity for hemorrhaging.

Manifestations of bleeding in PV can differ in location and severity. Gums, the epidermis, the nose (epistaxis), and the gastrointestinal tract are all frequent locations of hemorrhage. Hematuria (blood in the urine) or excessive menstrual hemorrhage in women may also manifest in certain individuals. Although minor bleeding episodes may not demand medical intervention, severe or recurrent bleeding may warrant the use of blood transfusions or platelet-lowering therapies.

Splenomegaly, Or Spleen Enlargement, In Polycythemia Vera

An enlarged spleen, or splenomegaly, is a frequent complication of PV. The filtration of blood and elimination of faulty or decrepit blood cells are functions performed by the spleen. Increased erythrocyte production in PV may result in splenic enlargement due to the spleen's increased workload in processing the surplus cells.

Symptoms associated with enlarged spleen in PV include abdominal pain or discomfort, early satiety, and a sensation of fullness in the abdomen. An enlarged spleen may occasionally be identified via imaging studies, including computed tomography (CT) scans or physical examinations. The primary objectives of splenomegaly management in PV are typically symptom relief and treatment of the underlying condition. Medication or surgical excision (splenectomy) to reduce the bulk of the spleen may be considered in certain instances.

The Occurrence Of Myelofibrosis In Polycythemia Vera

Myelofibrosis is a progressive disorder of the bone marrow in which fibrous scar tissue replaces healthy bone marrow.

In contrast to PV, which is distinguished by an excessive generation of red blood cells, myelofibrosis may manifest as a subsequent complication of PV or other MPNs. Although the precise mechanisms that contribute to myelofibrosis development in PV remain unknown, it is hypothesized that they involve the aberrant proliferation of blood cells and the secretion of inflammatory cytokines.

Progressive myelofibrosis may manifest in PV, accompanied by anemia, fatigue, splenomegaly, and an elevated vulnerability to infections. A bone marrow biopsy is commonly employed to validate the diagnosis of myelofibrosis in PV, as it detects the existence of fibrosis and other distinctive alterations.

The primary objective of myelofibrosis management in PV is symptom alleviation. This may involve the administration of supportive care, medications to control anemia or other complications, and, in certain instances, stem cell transplantation.

CHAPTER FOUR

Transformation Of Leukemia In Polycythemia Vera

While PV is classified as a chronic condition, acute leukemia, specifically acute myeloid leukemia (AML), remains a potential complication. Leukemia transformation in PV is characterized by the progression of genetic mutations within the aberrant blood cells, which results in unrestrained proliferation and compromised differentiation. Although the incidence of leukemia transformation in PV is comparatively uncommon, it does escalate as the disease progresses and in conjunction with specific risk factors, including advanced age or a prior occurrence of blood clotting.

It is critical to monitor for indications of leukemia transformation when managing PV. Leukemia transformation may manifest as fatigue, weight loss that cannot be explained, fever, the propensity for easy injury or bleeding, and recurrent infections. The confirmation of a leukemia transformation diagnosis generally requires the utilization of bone marrow biopsy and genetic testing. Leukemia transformation in PV may be managed through targeted therapy, stem cell transplantation, or intensive chemotherapy, contingent upon factors such as the patient's age, general health, and particular genetic mutations.

Treatment For Polycythemia Vera

While enhancing quality of life, PV management seeks to reduce the risk of complications such as blood clotting, hemorrhage episodes, and myelofibrosis. Essential elements of PV management include:

1. Phlebotomy: When PV is initially diagnosed, routine blood removal (phlebotomy) is performed to reduce blood viscosity and the risk of

blood clotting. Phlebotomy procedures may be conducted at consistent time intervals until the hematocrit levels fall within the desired range.

2. Medications: Phlebotomy may be accompanied by the prescription of medications to reduce the risk of complications and regulate blood cell production. Hypoxic agents such as hydroxyurea, interferon-alpha, and JAK2 inhibitors like ruxolitinib are frequently prescribed to treat PV.

3. Aspirin Therapy: In patients with PV who have a low to moderate risk of cardiovascular events, low-dose aspirin may be prescribed to reduce the risk of blood clotting.

4. Consistent surveillance of vital signs, symptoms, and the advancement of the disease is imperative to efficiently manage PV. This may entail routine laboratory assessments, imaging investigations, and clinical evaluations.

5. Lifestyle Modifications: By embracing a healthy lifestyle, which encompasses consistent physical activity, maintaining healthy body weight, and abstaining from tobacco and excessive alcohol usage, the likelihood of complications can be diminished and overall health can be enhanced.

6. Sustained Care: To manage symptoms such as fatigue, pruritus, or splenomegaly, it may be necessary to administer supportive care interventions, such as pharmacotherapy, to mitigate distress or enhance overall well-being.

7. Patient Education: It is critical to offer education and support to individuals with PV and their families to encourage treatment adherence, facilitate the identification of potential complications, and empower them to make well-informed decisions regarding their healthcare.

In summary, Polycythemia Vera necessitates all-encompassing treatment to mitigate the likelihood of complications and enhance overall well-being. A comprehensive comprehension of PV, encompassing its multifaceted manifestations such as splenomegaly, myelofibrosis, leukemia transformation, and efficacious management strategies, enables healthcare practitioners to deliver individualized care to patients. Ongoing investigations into the fundamental mechanisms of PV and the formulation of innovative treatment strategies offer the potential for further enhancing the prognosis for those impacted by this uncommon ailment.

Continued Care

Consistent post-diagnostic follow-up care is imperative to monitor the advancement of the condition and effectively manage symptoms after the diagnosis of PV. Contingent to the presence of complications and the severity of the condition, the frequency of follow-up appointments may differ.

In general, once a patient's condition has stabilized, they are advised to visit their healthcare provider every few months; thereafter, the frequency of visits should decrease.

During subsequent visits, medical professionals may conduct a range of evaluations, which may consist of:

1. A physical examination serves the purpose of assessing the patient's general well-being and identifying any indications of disease advancement or complications.

2. Routine blood tests are essential for the monitoring of various blood counts, such as platelet count, white blood cell count, and red blood cell count.

These examinations aid in determining the efficacy of treatments and identify any irregularities that might necessitate intervention.

3. Bone Marrow Biopsy: A bone marrow biopsy may be required in certain instances to assess the response to treatment and determine the extent of bone marrow involvement.

4. Imaging Studies: Complications such as blood clotting or organ involvement may be identified using imaging techniques such as ultrasound, CT, or MRI.

5. Symptom Assessment: During follow-up visits, patients should inform their healthcare provider of any newly developed or worsening symptoms, as timely intervention may be necessary to effectively manage them.

Counting Blood Via Monitoring

Blood count monitoring is an essential component of PV management, as it facilitates the evaluation of disease progression and informs treatment choices. The principal blood components that are monitored are:

1. Red Blood Cell Count (RBC): PV is characterized by an elevated RBC count. Frequent assessment of red blood cell (RBC) count aids in determining the extent of erythrocytosis and influences treatment choices, including phlebotomy or medication administration.

2. White Blood Cell Count (WBC): While less frequent than erythrocytosis, an elevated WBC count may occur in some cases of PV. WBC count monitoring aids in the identification of abnormalities and indicators of disease progression.

3. Platelet Count: An increased production of blood cells in the bone marrow may result in an elevated platelet count in PV. Platelet count monitoring facilitates the evaluation of thrombosis risk and informs treatment decisions.

4. Hematocrit level, denoted as Hct, indicates the percentage of total blood volume that is composed of red blood cells. PV is characterized by elevated hematocrit levels, which are closely monitored to determine the severity of the disease and direct treatment.

Initially, routine blood tests are typically conducted every few weeks; once the disease has reached a stable state, they are conducted less frequently. Nevertheless, the frequency of monitoring may differ based on patient-specific variables and the response to treatment.

CHAPTER FIVE

Complementary Therapies

Consistent with targeted interventions that concentrate on symptom management and blood cell count reduction, supportive therapies are of paramount importance in the administration of PV. The aforementioned treatments are designed to mitigate complications, enhance overall well-being, and cater to the distinct requirements of every individual. The following are some supportive therapies for PV:

1.   Phlebotomy, alternatively referred to as bloodletting, is the principal therapeutic approach for PV to diminish blood cell counts and blood viscosity. A specific volume of blood is extracted from the body via venipuncture during phlebotomy to reduce hematocrit levels and avert complications like blood clotting.

2. Medication Therapy: Symptoms associated with PV, including fatigue, irritation, and enlarged spleen (splenomegaly), may be treated with prescribed medications. Prominent pharmaceutical agents employed in the management of PV comprise ruxolitinib, interferon-alpha, hydroxyurea, and aspirin.

3. Anticoagulant Therapy: Patients diagnosed with PV are at a heightened risk of developing blood clots; therefore, they may be prescribed low-dose anticoagulants or anticoagulant medications (e.g., aspirin) to mitigate the potential for thrombotic events (e.g., stroke or heart attack).

4. Patients with PV must ensure they maintain adequate hydration to prevent the formation of blood clots and enhance blood flow. Patients are frequently advised to avoid dehydration by consuming copious amounts of fluids, especially water.

5. Lifestyle Modifications: Patients with PV can effectively manage symptoms and reduce the risk of complications by adopting a healthy lifestyle. This may encompass engaging in consistent physical activity, sustaining a healthy body weight, abstaining from tobacco use, and adhering to a well-balanced dietary regimen that is abundant in whole cereals, fruits, and vegetables.

Early prognosis

PV prognoses vary based on several variables, including the age at which the condition manifests, the presence or absence of complications, the patient's response to treatment, and their overall health. Many patients with PV can lead relatively normal lives and have a life expectancy close to the norm when treated appropriately.

However, PV is associated with an increased risk of prognostic-altering complications such as stroke, heart attack, and blood clotting. As a result of inadequate treatment or management, the likelihood of complications increases in cases of PV.

In addition, PV has the potential to develop into more severe myeloproliferative neoplasms, including acute myeloid leukemia and myelofibrosis, both of which have the potential to impact the prognosis.

Consistent monitoring and compliance with treatment guidelines are critical to maximize prognosis and reduce the likelihood of complications in individuals diagnosed with PV.

The Expectancy Of Life

Recent years have witnessed a substantial increase in the life expectancy of patients with PV due to developments in diagnosis and treatment. After diagnosis, many patients with PV can expect to live for decades with proper management.

The life expectancy of patients diagnosed with PV may be influenced by a multitude of factors, which encompass:

1. Life expectancy may be reduced in older patients with PV as a result of comorbidities and an elevated susceptibility to complications, including cardiovascular events.

2. The existence of complications: Life expectancy can be substantially affected by the development of complications, including thrombosis, hemorrhage, or progression to more advanced forms of myeloproliferative neoplasms.

3. The prognosis for patients is generally more favorable when they attain excellent disease control and respond positively to treatment, as

opposed to those who do not exhibit a satisfactory response to therapy.

4. The life expectancy of patients with PV may also be impacted by their overall health status and the prevalence of any additional medical conditions.

5. Ensuring Treatment Adherence: It is critical for patients diagnosed with PV to comply with treatment recommendations, which encompass routine blood monitoring and lifestyle adjustments, to maximize outcomes and extend life expectancy.

In general, although PV is a chronic condition necessitating lifelong management, with proper treatment and routine monitoring, a considerable number of patients can anticipate a comparatively typical lifespan. For patients with PV to achieve optimal outcomes and increase their life expectancy, close collaboration between patients and healthcare providers is vital.

Future Directions And Research In Polycythemia Vera

Notwithstanding the progress made in comprehending the etiology and management of PV, there are still numerous domains that warrant investigation to enhance scientific comprehension and improve patient outcomes:

1. Further investigation into the molecular mechanisms that govern the development and progression of PV is crucial to discovering innovative therapeutic targets and biomarkers. Investigations that center on genetic mutations, signaling pathways, and the microenvironment of the bone marrow can yield significant knowledge regarding the pathogenesis of PV.

2. Risk stratification is an important aspect of PV, as it enables the development of more accurate prognostications and facilitates the implementation of personalized treatment strategies for thrombotic

and hemorrhagic complications. The integration of clinical, genetic, and biomarker data has the potential to inform therapeutic decision-making and improve risk prediction.

3. Exploring Innovative Therapeutic Agents: The exploration of novel therapeutic agents, such as immunomodulatory agents and targeted therapies, exhibits the potential to enhance treatment effectiveness and mitigate toxicity in PV. Clinical trials are currently in progress to assess the safety and effectiveness of novel pharmaceuticals, including interferon-based therapies, JAK inhibitors, and histone deacetylase inhibitors.

4. The optimization of therapeutic outcomes in PV may be achieved by adopting a precision medicine approach that takes into account individual patient characteristics, such as genetic profile, disease phenotype, and treatment response. The objective of precision medicine approaches is to customize treatment plans according to the specific

requirements of every patient, to optimize effectiveness while reducing untoward consequences.

5. The integration of patient-reported outcomes (PROs) into clinical practice and research can yield significant insights regarding the effects of PV on patients' treatment preferences and quality of life. By evaluating PROs such as symptom burden, quality of life, and treatment satisfaction, therapeutic objectives can be prioritized and patient-centered care can be enhanced.

In summary, continuous scientific endeavors that concentrate on molecular pathogenesis, risk stratification, innovative therapeutics, precision medicine, and patient-reported outcomes are indispensable for the progression of photovoltaic research and the future enhancement of patient outcomes.

CHAPTER SIX

Experimental Clinics For Polycythemia Vera

Clinical trials are of paramount importance in the progression of knowledge and therapeutic interventions for polycythemia vera (PV). The objective of these investigations is to assess the tolerability, effectiveness, and safety of innovative therapeutic agents, treatment approaches, and supportive care interventions. Principal components of clinical trials in PV include:

1. Therapeutic Targets: In PV clinical trials, a range of objectives are frequently pursued, encompassing the prevention of thrombotic events, mitigation of symptoms, enhancement of quality of life, and reduction of elevated red blood cell counts.

2. Clinical trials in PV may utilize observational studies, randomized controlled trials (RCTs), phase I-IV trials, registry studies, and observational studies, among others. For establishing the safety and efficacy of novel treatments in comparison to placebo or standard therapies, RCTs are especially crucial.

3. Endpoints: Hematologic response (e.g., hematocrit level normalization), reduction in thrombotic events, amelioration of symptom burden, and overall survival are typical endpoints in PV clinical trials.

In PV trials, patient-reported outcomes (PROs), including quality of life (QoL) metrics, are becoming an increasing number of acknowledged endpoints.

4. The selection of participants for PV clinical trials generally entails adherence to eligibility criteria, which encompass particular diagnostic

standards, disease stage, age limitations, and the exclusion of patients with substantial comorbidities or previous exposure to specific treatments. Diverse patient populations are incorporated to increase the generalizability of study results.

5. Ethical Considerations: Clinical trials involving PV must adhere to principles of ethics, which encompass safeguarding participant rights, ensuring transparency in study conduct, obtaining informed consent, and undergoing rigorous supervision by regulatory authorities and institutional review boards (IRBs).

6. The design, implementation, and dissemination of clinical trials in PV are facilitated through the collaborative endeavors of academic institutions, pharmaceutical companies, patient advocacy organizations, and regulatory agencies operating at multiple centers.

The inclusion of multiple sites in multicenter trials improves patient recruitment, diversity, and the generalizability of findings.

7. Clinical Practice Translation: The advancement of evidence-based guidelines, treatment algorithms, and regulatory approvals for novel therapies is facilitated by the success of clinical trials in PV. When trial results are incorporated into clinical practice, patient care and outcomes are enhanced.

In conclusion, clinical trials play a critical role in furthering knowledge and developing treatments for PV, substantiating the efficacy of innovative therapies, and enhancing patient outcomes. For PV clinical research to be successful, stakeholder collaboration, adherence to ethical standards, and the translation of trial results into clinical practice are indispensable.

Progress In The Management Of Polycythemia Vera

Progress in the management of polycythemia vera (PV) has revolutionized the approach to this chronic myeloproliferative neoplasm by concentrating on symptom control, thrombotic complication reduction, and quality of life enhancement. Notable developments encompass:

1. Phlebotomy, which involves the removal of surplus blood, continues to be a fundamental component of photovoltaic (PV) therapy to mitigate increased hematocrit levels and the potential for thrombosis. The implementation of individualized phlebotomy protocols is beneficial in regulating hematocrit levels within desired ranges and mitigating symptoms.

2. Cytoreductive Therapy: In high-risk PV patients, cytoreductive therapy attempts to inhibit bone marrow hyperactivity and reduce the

risk of thrombotic events. As a cytoreducing agent administered orally, hydroxyurea is frequently employed as a primary therapeutic approach to regulate platelet counts and avert thrombosis. Busulfan and interferon-alpha are substitute cytoreductive agents that can be administered to patients who exhibit intolerance or resistance to hydroxyurea.

3. The introduction of innovative therapeutic agents, specifically Janus kinase (JAK) inhibitors, has broadened the range of treatment alternatives available to patients with PV. Ruxolitinib, a JAK1/JAK2 inhibitor, has exhibited effectiveness in patients with symptomatic splenomegaly and inadequate response to or intolerance to hydroxyurea by reducing spleen size, controlling symptoms, and enhancing quality of life.

4. Antithrombotic therapy is of paramount importance in PC patients who have a prior thrombotic event or possess high-risk

characteristics, as it effectively mitigates the risk of thrombotic complications. For primary thromboprophylaxis in PV, low-dose aspirin is advised as first-line therapy; in high-risk patients, cytoreductive therapy with hydroxyurea or interferon-alpha may be administered.

5. Risk stratification is a management approach that involves the use of a revised International Prognostic Scoring System (IPSS-R) and International Prognostic Score of Thrombosis in Essential Thrombocythemia (IPSET-thrombosis) models. These models assist in the identification of patients with PV who are at a heightened risk of thrombosis and could potentially derive advantages from more aggressive therapeutic measures, such as cytoreductive therapy and antithrombotic prophylaxis.

6. Supportive Care: Essential components of PV treatment are supportive care measures, which include the management of symptoms such as

fatigue, pruritus, and microvascular disturbances. Anxiety reduction, symptom management, lifestyle adjustments, and psychological assistance all contribute to enhanced patient health and quality of life.

7. Combination therapy, which involves the use of cytoreductive agents and JAK inhibitors, may offer synergistic advantages for patients with PV who do not respond adequately to single-agent therapy or develop intolerance to them, according to emerging evidence. Ongoing clinical trials are assessing combination regimens to maximize treatment efficacy and minimize adverse effects.

In summary, the management of PV has been significantly transformed by therapeutic developments such as phlebotomy, cytoreductive therapy, novel agents including JAK inhibitors, antithrombotic therapy, risk stratification, supportive care, and combination therapy. These advancements have resulted in improved patient outcomes and quality of life. Continuous investigation and cooperation among pharmaceutical companies, clinicians, and researchers will persist in propelling innovation and refining treatment approaches for PV.

Summary

In summary, Polycythemia Vera (PV) is a persistent and potentially fatal hematological condition distinguished by an excessive synthesis of erythrocytes within the bone marrow. PV is a complex condition requiring vigilant monitoring and management to avert complications including blood clotting, strokes, and heart attacks, despite its apparent simplicity.

Efforts to reduce the risk of coagulation while managing symptoms and complications are the goals of PV treatment. Pharmaceutical approaches frequently incorporate routine blood draws (phlebotomy) to reduce the hematocrit level, in addition to pharmacological interventions that impede thrombus formation or the production of blood cells.

Notwithstanding the progress made in comprehending PV and its therapeutic approaches, there continue to be obstacles in efficiently managing the ailment. There is a potential for patients to encounter symptoms that hurt their quality of life, as well as a chance that the disease may advance or evolve into more severe blood disorders.

Further investigation is being conducted to elucidate the fundamental mechanisms of PV and examine innovative therapeutic strategies. Furthermore, patient education and support play a pivotal role in enabling individuals with PV to take an active role in their treatment and develop well-informed choices regarding their health.

At its core, despite the considerable obstacles posed by Polycythemia Vera, individuals afflicted with this condition can achieve personal satisfaction and mitigate the hazards associated with the disorder through the implementation of appropriate medical treatment, management, and support.

THE END